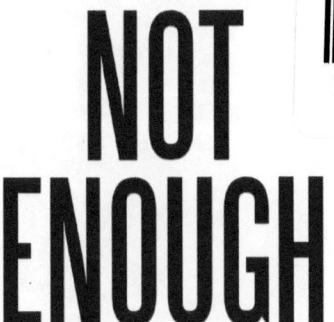

NOT ENOUGH

The Journey To Improve Overall Health and Kidney Function with Proper Diet Changes, Stem Cell Treatments, Acupuncture, And the Desire To Avoid Dialysis

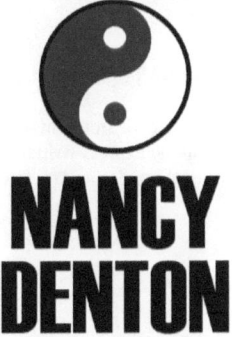

NANCY DENTON

outskirtspress

DENVER, COLORADO

Not Enough
The Journey To Improve Overall Health And Kidney Function With Proper Diet Changes, Stem Cell Treatments, Acupuncture, And The Desire To Avoid Dialysis
All Rights Reserved.
Copyright © 2014 Nancy Denton
v3.0

Outskirts Press, Inc.
http://www.outskirtspress.com

ISBN: 978-1-4787-3327-0

Outskirts Press and the "OP" logo are trademarks belonging to Outskirts Press, Inc.

PRINTED IN THE UNITED STATES OF AMERICA

"When they start kicking dirt in your face, you'll do whatever you have to do to stay around a while".

—Jim's thoughts on how to "stick with" strict dietary changes when your medical condition(s) require it for stabilization.

*"We only get to dance through life once;
when the tune changes, we just
have to change our dance routine".*

—Author's thoughts on how
to make lifestyle changes
when your health status
changes.

FOREWORD

Most of us try to do everything we can to stay relatively healthy. In spite of our best efforts, things go wrong. The causes may be hereditary, lifestyle choices, diet, etc. We do all the things we are told to make a difference; stop nicotine/smoking, stop drinking alcoholic beverages, drink the proper amount of water every day, stop using salt, adhere to a strict diet, take the medications prescribed to us by our doctor, and get proper rest/sleep. Yet, despite our best efforts, the lab results and tests continue to show a decline. Slowly, but still a decline. We watch others we know with the same health issues that continue down the road of unhealthy habits and lifestyles, yet they do not decline in the same way. We want to throw up our hands and say forget it. But, we know the alternative is not what we want. We are all different, inside and out. The kidneys are just one example of this. There are people who do not worry about keeping their blood pressure, blood sugar, stress levels, etc. in what are considered healthy ranges. Their kidneys seem fine, while others who strive to do all the right things continue down the road to kidney failure. And the same can apply to many illnesses.

ACKNOWLEDGMENT

I dedicate this book to my loving, kind, hard-working husband, Jim. Through this journey, he has continued to work hard every day. He works in the physically and mentally challenging profession of construction, building beautiful homes, remodeling, etc. Jim makes happen exactly what the customer wants. He knows and understands all phases and aspects of construction from start to finish, with an eye for detail like no other. He keeps going, even through the days of feeling tired, and gets frustrated with the decline in his endurance. Jim calls it," having trouble staying hooked up".

PURPOSE

I started this book with the intent of writing a cookbook to help others with kidney disease maintain stable lab results by following a healthy diet; to keep the kidneys functioning without having to start dialysis, or for those on dialysis to stay healthier.

As our journey progresses, I realize there's so much more knowledge to share. I have been a Registered Nurse for 28 years. Always teaching others about disease management, diets, medications, signs and symptoms to report, and questions to ask their doctor. I was trained to approach nursing as a holistic concept; because to just start and administer an intravenous fluid or medication, perform wound care, provide care to a ventilator, surgical, cardiac, cancer, Alzheimer's, and patients from all walks of life, is only a small part of helping others move toward a healthier state of being. For example, if a person has a wound and they are nutritionally compromised; the wound very likely will not heal.

INTRODUCTION

There are many cookbooks and recipes that address diabetes and cooking sugar free. You can find information on diabetic and renal diets readily available. Many people that do not have diabetes may have low kidney function because of high blood pressure. The mindset in much of mainstream medicine today is that a person can eat anything, just in moderation, regardless of their diagnosis or disease processes.

I am writing this book to help people better understand what they can eat with low kidney function, diabetes, or hypertension because many people look at the long list of what not to eat, and think, "What else is there"? "I can't eat anything". Part of the dilemma is cultural, depending on where you're from and what you're used to eating. Here in Northeast Oklahoma, many people grow up eating brown beans, fried potatoes, corn bread or biscuits and most meats are always fried. These foods are still a favorite meal for many in this region.

I have been a registered nurse for 28 years, acquiring experience in different areas, but always teaching patients and families about disease processes, diets, and how to care for themselves or loved ones. And yes, I did practice what I preach in my own home. I did not raise my children with quick, easy junk foods, sweets, or sodas. These were a rare treat for my family.

So, following a diabetic diet was what I was used to, even though I am not diabetic. Jim was good about his diet, and he was never ill. He did not go to the doctor very much at all. I conveyed to him that he should have an annual checkup even though he felt good. We both went for our annual check ups in October, 2010, and Jim's lab results came back showing his glomelular filtration rate (GFR), which shows the percentage of kidney function, at 23 percent. The physician also told Jim he more than likely had a blood pressure in the lower end of the high range for quite some time. Jim was started on a blood pressure medication, and a referral was made to a nephrologist (kidney specialist) of our choice. Jim had been a diabetic for 19 years at that point, taking good care of himself, and still working in construction every day; and still does to this day!

During our first visit to the nephrologist, we were handed a thick manila envelope and told, "Here is some good information and recipes". We read through the literature, and did not find it very helpful. Jim's lab results the next month showed his GFR at 21 percent, with following a strict diabetic diet. With my nursing knowledge and experience, our own in-depth research, more reading, clinical visits with a registered dietitian that I knew for years through working with her, and discussions with Jim's nephrologist during his appointments, we armed ourselves with the knowledge and mindset to achieve Jim's goal of never having to start renal dialysis.

This has only been accomplished by adhering to a strict diet. I adhere to the same diet, which makes it easier for Jim. I have experimented with baking desserts, cooking meats, etc. Learning how to make it all taste good has been a challenge. We read ALL food labels while shopping for groceries. This is a must! We look for sugar, carbohydrate, potassium, phosphate, and fat content of all foods; pasta, cereal, sauces,...

My goal is to help others know what they can eat and drink, without having to wade through the long list of " no-no" foods and drinks, or the foods with very limited amounts allowed. I hope to simplify all this so eating at home or eating out can be enjoyable. After all, variety is supposed to be the "spice of life".

OUTLINE

CHAPTER 1

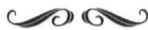

NOT ENOUGH TIME

The flight schedule was going to be a challenge. We only had two hours on the ground between each flight, and with Jim's poor endurance, shortness of breath, and continued left ankle pain, it was not enough time. The only hope for getting from flight to flight with international travel was to request a wheelchair and escort at every airport. Jim's health motivated us to make a decision outside our comfort zone. Jim's kidney function was not improving.

Our body filters toxins from our bloodstream by the liver and kidneys. The toxins that are excreted by the kidneys pass through a membrane from the renal artery to the filters in the kidneys. These filters are usually what gets scarred or damaged and no longer function properly. There are people that can get improved kidney function with moderate dietary adjustments and proper medication, while others, no matter how stringent their diet and life-style changes, get little or no improvement in their health.

Most people have two kidneys. One on each side, located just below, or at the bottom of the rib cage in the lumbar region of the back. Each kidney is approximately 4 inches long, 2 inches wide, 1 inch thick, and weighs about 4 to 6 ounces. Each kidney functions to filter the blood, excreting the end products of body metabolism in the form of urine, and regulating the concentration of hydrogen, sodium, potassium, phosphate, and other ions in the extra-cellular fluid. (A general term for all the body fluids outside the cells).

Kidney disease can take on many forms and have many causes. Kidney failure can be caused by acute or chronic processes, and the result can be complete loss of kidney function. The toxins normally eliminated by the kidneys accumulates in the body fluids as a result of impaired renal excretion and leads to a disruption in homeostatic, endocrine, and metabolic functions. Kidney failure is a disease affecting the entire body. This can result in poor endurance, shortness of breath, low energy, decreased strength, and many other symptoms that may become discouraging to people.

CHAPTER 2

❧ ❧

NOT ENOUGH INFORMATION

I asked Jim to allow me to schedule him an appointment for an annual examination by his physician. The man never slowed down long enough to take time for such things. Jim said he always felt good. The words of a true workaholic.

The news we received after that appointment was shocking. Although Jim had been a diabetic for years, he tried to take care of himself by eating right, taking his insulin, and managing his overall health and stress levels well. Jim's kidney function was at 23 percent!

Jim asked the doctor how this could happen, but there just wasn't enough information to make that determination since he was now showing an elevated blood pressure also. Jim said as far as he knew that was never a problem before.

Jim and I were three months into our new relationship when all this happened, so we began our journey of love and life together. Jim would ask questions; I would share my knowledge, and we would seek more information on ways to improve Jim's health.

Acute kidney failure can be reversible, depending on cause and the body's ability to heal. Some causes may be trauma, medications toxic to the kidneys, infection, severe dehydration, etc.

Chronic kidney failure is a slower process, causing the kidneys to lose the ability to filter toxins out of the body. There can be some improvement, depending on what has caused the problem such as a blockage can be repaired, improvement in blood pressure or blood sugar control or stopping medications (only with a physician's order).

With chronic kidney disease (CKD), there are five stages. Stage V (ESRD), or end-stage renal disease, is usually when dialysis is started. The GFR as seen on lab results is usually at or below 15. The GFR indicates the percentage of kidney function that is remaining.

CHAPTER 3

❦

NOT ENOUGH RESOURCES

As Jim's kidney function declined, despite all of our efforts, including four months of consultations with Julia, a registered dietitian that I've known for years, massive research on diet changes, discussions with Jim's nephrologist, our continued strict diet, and more research; we had to make a decision to stay the course and prepare for dialysis or join the ranks opting for alternative treatment options. Jim's goal is to never have to start dialysis.

After two years of research and a discussion with the nephrologist, Jim made the decision to go for stem cell treatments in Thailand.

The cost was expensive, but compared to the cost of

dialysis or other treatments in the United States, the thought wasn't so mind-boggling. A friend, Helen Alewine, put it into perspective by saying, " If you needed a new car, you would not hesitate to sign a note for $30,000 dollars". And how true that is with the need to get back and forth to work every day, as we do not live or work in a metro area with public transportation.

We did not have enough resources readily available, so we refinanced our home. All was going well with the process. We had a closing date set, locked into a great fixed rate, and at the end of the week prior to the week of closing; the bank called and said it was decided that we needed to finish the new siding on the home. We were in the middle of this process when we decided to refinance. This was on Good Friday, and they wanted to take pictures of the completed project on Monday of the following week. Had it not been for the help of great friends and family, we could not have completed it because of Jim's low energy and poor endurance.

Our closing for the refinance took place on April 2, 2013, just three days before traveling to Thailand.

CHAPTER 4

⌒⌒ ⌒⌒

NOT ENOUGH CHOICES

Jim's physician made the referral to the nephrologist of our choice in Tahlequah. When we arrived at the first appointment, we were told Jim's doctor had to be out of town. Jim was asked if he would see the new nephrologist in the office, and he agreed.

She requested, and wrote an order for multiple lab tests to be done within one week of our next appointment. Three weeks later we were at the Tahlequah laboratory, and with Jim not having health insurance at that time, the cost was $1200 dollars, payable that day! A week later, we went to Jim's second appointment with the new nephrologist where she reviewed all the lab results. She stated she would like to schedule a CT scan with contrast of Jim's kidneys to make a differential diagnosis as to the cause of Jim's kidney disease. She cautioned Jim that the contrast may well put him into complete kidney failure and he would be started on dialysis if that were the case.

Prior to leaving the doctor's office, we asked the receptionist to make Jim's future appointments with our first choice/request for a nephrologist.

Over the next two weeks, Jim and I discussed it, and then discussed it with his primary care physician. Jim decided not to have the scan, and I canceled the appointment two days prior to his going.

Jim's choice for a nephrologist, at my recommendation, was honored on his third visit. We explained to this nephrologist that we cancelled the CT scan with contrast due to the concern of a high probability of putting Jim into complete kidney failure. The nephrologist stated it more than likely would have done this. At that point, I asked if he would consider an ultrasound of the kidneys, and he agreed and ordered the test.

The nephrologist asked Jim if he would agree to dialysis, if and when the time comes. Jim told the doctor, "Yes, I would like to be around a while".

The nurse handed us a thick manila envelope and said, " There is some good information and recipes in there, and it would be better if you didn't have dairy products".

During subsequent visits, the nephrologist discussed the pros and cons of kidney transplant, various types of dialysis, and dialysis treatments in a center or at home. Jim and I made the decision for home dialysis if the need occurs, but Jim continues to remind them of his goal to NEVER have to start dialysis. I offered Jim one of my kidneys for transplant, if I would be a match, but he chose not to explore having this as the risk for complications or death is high related to the anti-rejection drugs needed after receiving a donor kidney, potential infections, and numerous other postoperative complications that could occur.

CHAPTER 5

❦

NOT ENOUGH TREATMENT OPTIONS

During the ongoing process of doctor visits, monthly labs, adjusting our diet based on the lab results, and managing symptoms of Jim's blood pressure and blood sugar changes with phone calls to doctors, our research for new or better treatment options continued. Through it all we continue to work full-time jobs every day, before and after our journey.

Jim made the statement that he has been surprised and saddened by his experience because he thought all doctors would do whatever was necessary to make a person better. He now feels that our main-stream medical model is to, " Treat my symptoms and get me ready for dialysis, not try to heal me".

Jim says he wants to feel good and stay active. Although this may be possible on dialysis, the risk of complications or adverse effects is great, especially with long-term dialysis.

Jim's nephrologist recommended Jim have a surgical procedure to create a Cimino fistula in his left wrist so it could mature and be ready if the need for dialysis arises. We were told the risk of dying from an infection goes up 40% if a central line would need to be inserted for dialysis. As a registered nurse, I know this to be true. Especially with methicillin resistant staph aereus (MRSA) infections becoming the "norm" and not the exception in this day and time.

During our two years of research, we explored clinical trials, the process of stem cell treatment in the United States, and looked at/ read many research papers and the research results. Stem cell treatments, using autologous (your own), or donor stem cells, administered intravenously without wiping out the immune system, is not a treatment modality approved by the FDA. Many nations of the world are offering, and providing, these treatments with great success for many illnesses or disease processes, but not our country.

It is called medical tourism. Most of the stories you

read or hear about are the horror stories. There are many more positive success stories. Many celebrities have been to other countries for treatments or surgeries. Some thoughts on this subject are that our pharmaceutical giants and health insurance companies are the driving forces behind health care policies in our great nation so they can continue with profits in the millions year after year. We believe in free enterprise, but also believe more could be done to heal people, not just treat symptoms.

Jim's options were to get on the kidney transplant list, and/or prepare for dialysis. Jim opted to travel to Thailand, (both of us), and receive stem cell treatments and acupuncture. He was given the choice of using his own stem cells or donor stem cells. Jim chose donor stem cells that are extracted from baby teeth, after a young child loses them.

Dr. Kampon Sriwatanakul's belief and theory about not wiping out the immune system prior to administering stem cells is: "If you have a few bad people in town, you do not wipe them out, you bring in more good people to change the environment".

A comment made by a colleague is, "Here in the United States, the prevalence of a physician or medical facility being sued is so great, even if the treatment went well, but the results did not last as long as a person thought it should, is a possible reason for the climate in the medical community".

Many people, including persons in the medical field are returning to natural remedies, herbal preparations, acupuncture, and fresh foods or vegan diets. While in Thailand for treatments, the physicians worked with us to improve Jim's diet even more. This is to be a permanent lifestyle change.

CHAPTER 6

⫘

NOT ENOUGH NUTRITION

The renal component of Jim's diet is definitely the most challenging. There are many views on what people should eat to maintain a healthy diet. For a healthy person stable weight is a good reflection of their diet. For a person with diabetes, stable blood sugars and stable weight would be the goal. For a person with high blood pressure (hypertension) or cardiac diagnosis, stable blood pressure readings, stable weight, and cholesterol levels within normal limits would be ideal. A person can have many health challenges occurring at the same time such as diabetes, high blood pressure, low kidney function, arthritis, and of course there are many more that could be listed. Most disease processes would allow and benefit from a typical vegetarian diet, or just a reduction in red meat and concentrated sweets or sugars from the diet, but not so with the renal diet. The renal diet consists of foods to avoid, limit, and some that are never to be eaten. This is because low functioning kidneys have difficulty filtering or allowing reabsorption in some cases of potassium, phosphates, proteins, and other nutrients.

The theory with eliminating all meat from the diet, except fish and some seafood such as shrimp or crabmeat, is to make Jim's diet more alkaline. A more acidic pH in our body attributes to an increase in inflammation. The Thai physicians believed, as seen on bio scan, Jim had inflammation everywhere, including the areas where toxins are moved from the blood, renal arteries, to the urinay system at the glomelular filters. With less inflammation comes improved functional processes internally which can equate to improved kidney function.

It is difficult to prevent iron deficient anemia, especially when a person with low kidney function follows a vegetarian diet because he or she has difficulty eating enough iron rich foods with the dietary restrictions. Foods rich in iron include beef or chicken liver, clams or muscles, oysters, cooked beef, sardines, cooked turkey, halibut, haddock, perch, salmon, tuna, ham, veal, lentils, beans, spinach, tofu, dried apricots, baked potato, broccoli, enriched egg noodles, wheat germ, some nuts, and there are more. From the above list, a person on a renal diet would be allowed the fish, (if it is not a fish with a potential for higher levels of mercury), seafood, limited spinach, broccoli, egg noodles, some beef, chicken, or turkey. Then to reduce inflammation, eliminate the beef, chicken, and turkey. As the Thai physicians stated, it isn't necessarily the meat but the hormones, antibiotics, and preservatives in the meats that are harmful.

As Jim's iron levels became low, I researched the possibility of finding a nutritional supplement that would aid in providing Jim enough iron in his diet. Iron tablets do not work as they are not well absorbed, and can cause gastrointestinal distress. In my research for a nutritional iron source, (I have many resource books at home and the use of the Internet), I read about the use of food source liquid iron. Jim and I drove to the closest health food store, OASIS, in Tahlequah. We spoke with Ellen, and she did not normally carry a product of this type, but she had just ordered some earlier in the week, which hadn't yet arrived. We reserved a large bottle of it with Ellen to call us as soon as it came in. This product has been the perfect solution as it is easily absorbed and has not caused

Jim any gastric distress. His only complaint is the taste, but he tolerates 10 ml every morning before breakfast. His monthly lab results show no signs of anemia. We have received many blessings in this journey, and food source liquid iron is one of them. The usual treatment for anemia in chronic kidney disease is intravenous iron infusions performed in a hospital as an outpatient procedure, when ordered by the nephrologist. To avoid the potential complications of infection, Jim prefers not to have intravenous iron infusions if at all possible.

We keep two food lists on the door of our refrigerator to remind us, always, of the foods to avoid or limit because of their potassium or phosphate content as high levels of potassium in the blood can cause cardiac arrhythmias or, if high enough, cardiac arrest, and high phosphate levels can result in hyperparathyroidism and osteodystrophy, resulting in bone disease which can make a person more prone to bone fractures.

With the kidney disease process, all potatoes should be leached,(soaked in water), for a few hours prior to cooking to reduce the potassium content. A great discovery has been canned sliced potatoes in water, low-sodium brand. After opening, rinse with water again. Of course, fresh is best for all fruits and vegetables, but low-sodium brands of canned or frozen vegetables is acceptable.

During the growing season for your area, the local farmers markets are usually a cost-effective means of obtaining fresh foods. If you meet the financial criteria for low income, most communities have food pantries that provide various food amounts based on family size. I teach patients that utilizing available resources that do not cost, helps toward having enough money to purchase other foods needed such as rice or almond milks to eliminate dairy from the diet, or veggie meat products on occasion, these are quite tasty.

These dietary changes are necessary, even if a person is on dialysis. It is a permanent life style change to maintain better health. A healthy diet, appropriate to an individual's needs, is absolutely crucial to achieving optimum health and longevity.

Do I adhere to this diet with my husband? Absolutely!

CHAPTER 7

∾⌾᪐

NOT ENOUGH PHYSICIAN ACCESS FOR CHANGES

Jim's blood pressure readings continued to stay in the 150s over the 80s, and his kidney function dropped 3% in one month. We were able to make an appointment with his primary care physician immediately. He added another blood pressure medication, and Jim's blood pressure decreased back to 130s over 60s and his kidney function is back to 22%.

Most nephrologists request their patients never start a new prescription medication or over-the-counter supplement/medication without their approval because they know whether or not it can be tolerated by the kidneys. Often, the problem comes in when the nephrologist is so busy that fitting in an extra appointment is nearly impossible. Any delay in adjusting or changing blood pressure medication, adding medication to counteract a high potassium or phosphate level, etc. can have detrimental or life-threatening consequences. A patient may end up in the emergency department of a hospital trying to explain his or her diagnosis, what medications they are on, symptoms, and try to get proper blood pressure management until they can see the nephrologist. Not to say a physician in the emergency department isn't a very knowledgeable person, but the needs of a person with chronic kidney disease is different than most as the liver and kidneys help to eliminate the waste by-products from eating, taking medications, and metabolism processes. There are physicians and other healthcare professionals that believe as long as the medication(s) somewhat controls the blood pressure, but causes edema of the lower extremities or other symptoms, it is still alright. I personally believe the only side effect you should have from a blood pressure medication is consistent blood pressure readings in the normal ranges of less than 140/80, or whatever your doctor deems is normal for you. There are more than enough medications to choose from, therefore it may take a few times to find the ones that work right for each individual.

I recommend a person with chronic kidney disease

maintain a primary care physician, a cardiologist, and a nephrologist so if problems occur, one of them should be able to see you quickly. This helps to maintain continuity of care. The patient's responsibility would be to share their information with all of their physicians, including each time one of them makes changes to the medication regimen. One should maintain an up-to-date medication list, and provide a copy to each physician, at every visit. It would be beneficial to carry a copy of this list in a purse or wallet at all times, and include allergies, diagnosis, type of diet your physician has ordered, name of physicians with phone numbers, and any special concern such as left wrist fistula (no labs, no blood pressures, do not use left arm for any type of medical access unless needed for dialysis); another example might be left chest port a cath, right chest central line/dual lumen; or if on dialysis state the type, frequency, and where administered with the facility phone number. This type of information can help prevent complications in an emergency and save your life.

Everyone should have, at a minimum, an annual physical examination with your primary care physician. During that visit to your physician some basic laboratory test (blood work) should be performed such as a Chem 12 or Chem 20 and a CBC. Some physician's offices draw labs and others send you to a local lab. The labs drawn will be based on your physician's orders with him/her taking into consideration any current disease processes, or new symptoms you may be experiencing. Depending on your health status, the frequency of physician visits and lab tests will be discussed with you by your doctor. Of course, all payments for medical care to health practitioners from Medicare, Medicaid, and private health insurance companies are based on medical necessity.

Some lab tests that will indicate to your physician the presence of kidney disease are the BUN and Creatinine. If those are abnormal he/she may order other lab tests that specifically look at your kidney function, such as a renal panel. These labs are generally not fasting labs unless your physician tells you differently. If you have a fistula or graft that has been surgically completed in preparation for hemodialysis, do not allow anyone to draw labs or perform blood pressure readings on that arm. This can cause blood clots or other damage/trauma and make your fistula or graft nonfunctional and unable to be used for dialysis.

I recommend you request a copy of all lab results from your physician each time labs are done and keep a medical file at your home. If you are on di-alysis in a clinic setting, such as Davita Dialysis or Fresenius Dialysis, these organizations have web-sites that can be accessed via computer/internet for viewing your lab results after you set up an account and log on. There is no charge for this service.

CHAPTER 8

❦

NOT ENOUGH READILY AVAILABLE INFORMATION FOR DIETARY ALTERNATIVES

After Jim's diagnosis of Stage IV Chronic Kidney Disease, he would want foods not allowed such as no bake cookies (no chocolate allowed), "real milk", and other food items. We researched and found health food stores, and visited them all in our search for alternative choices.

Within a few months of being told no meat, except fish and some seafood, Jim wanted a hamburger really bad. The hunt was on, and we found veggie meats.

Many health concerns, disease processes or illnesses, have special dietary needs to help a person improve or maintain their health status. A physician may order a diet appropriate to the needs of a person, based upon the medical diagnosis, medications being taken, food allergies or sensitivities, and laboratory results.

If a person is admitted in-patient status, at a medical facility, there will be a dietician and other dietary staff that can provide teaching and appropriate information for most diets. Where the problem lies, is not enough information about alternatives a person may use when told not to use chocolate, dairy or dairy products, red meat or no meats except fish, and some seafood, salt, and the list can go on and on.

This is when a person's hands go up and usually state, in frustration, "What else is left, what can I eat?" In reality, many people continue to eat the foods they shouldn't have because they are not usually aware of other choices.

We try not to use many soy products as these contain estrogens, which men have, but an imbalance of testosterone and estrogen hormones can occur. We found rice and almond milks, (the Thai physicians do not recommend coconut milk for diabetics); carob powder to replace chocolate; vegan cheeses (made from rice milk, almond milk, or soy); veggie meats (there are several brands available), some with soy and some without; green tea (dark-colored liquids are not recommended), but water is best, various flours for baking such as almond or rice (wheat flour products are not recommended by kidney professionals in the U.S., and white flour products are not recommended by the Thai physicians); and if you must have some salt to cook or eat, sea salt is recommended. We do not use salt to cook or use at the table. There are many great seasonings available to use for making dishes taste wonderful. Some of our favorites are Greek seasoning (sodium free), black pepper, garlic powder, lemon pepper, and turmeric. These can be used on any foods including eggs!

For those who do not live in a metropolitan area, the time, distance, and expense of driving to stores where many of the needed or desirable items are found is a deterrent in achieving better nutrition for improved health.

We spoke to the manager at our local supercenter. I requested some of the items that can now be purchased routinely such as rice and almond milk, veggie meats, and veggie cheese. We haven't accomplished getting the store to carry specialty flours, breads, or carob powder yet.

What we have found with many sugar-free products on the market is that they often cause intestinal bloating and gas related to the type of sugar substitute used. Through personal trial and error, we have found Stevia and Splenda to be the best tolerated. Of course, every individual is different with how various foods, sweeteners, spices, and fluids affect them. There are many articles and websites that discuss the negative side effects of sugar-free or natural sweeteners.

I have experimented with creating recipes to accomodate many health needs by using alternative food choices. It has been challenging, interesting, and hilarious at times. I continue doing this to give Jim interesting, flavorful choices in his/our diet. That will be my next writing project. A great cookbook to accommodate the dietary needs and choices of many people.

CHAPTER 9

⌒⌒⌒

IT'S NOT ENOUGH TO USE CONVENTIONAL DIABETIC RECIPES

With Jim's chronic kidney disease, the need to learn more about his special dietary needs was great. We followed a universally accepted diabetic diet, adhering to the exchange concept and no concentrated sweets, prior to his diagnosis of Stage IV Chronic Kidney Disease. Jim's kidney function continued to decline, even with the regimented, strict diet we followed for diabetic, hypertensive, renal disease.

At that time, we continued to eat beef, pork, chicken, and turkey meat products, but changed other things such as eliminating vegetables and fruits that are not recommended for a renal diet.

But we found that following standard recipes for hypertensive and diabetic diets was not enough. When the renal component was introduced into Jim's medical regimen, the old adage of "eat to live" became a reality. Learning the fine balance between proteins, fats (good versus unhealthy), carbohydrates, calories, food source vitamins, minerals and iron became such a challenge, that only through sheer determination and keeping Jim's goal of no dialysis foremost in our minds, have we successfully met his goal, still today.

A good example of a recipe for one of Jim's favorite occasional foods is No Bake Oatmeal Cookies. A standard diabetic recipe only changes regular granulated sugar to a sugar substitute. Now comes the renal component; no chocolate, no nuts, no peanut butter, and no dairy milk. We use quick oats, splenda, carob powder, and rice milk.. The recipe requires a longer cooking time (boiling) so the cookies will set up. Jim only gets these a couple times per year. Please don't ask how many batches I threw out before perfection for taste, texture, and looks was achieved!

To find frozen meals, for quick lunches or an occasional microwavable supper, without cheese from dairy, or without meats other than fish, shrimp, crabmeat, or occasional lobster has proven to be a challenge. Jim has these for lunch on workdays, and for the rare nights I'm not home due to mandatory nursing conferences associated with my work. He doesn't care for cooking.

There are recipes and recipe books available for diabetic diets that change up some ingredients to accommodate a few common allergies, which are very helpful, but not quite enough for the renal diet needs. There are some great websites for recipes and cookbooks that are specifically for the special needs of persons with renal disease. At www.kidneyhealth-gourmet.com, there is a cookbook newly updated July 2013, with some great recipes and information. My concern is that chicken, etc. will have antibiotics and/or hormones. Free range does not mean the absence of the above.

Most recipes can be easily changed to meet your dietary needs/restrictions. Once you learn, or keep a list, of your dietary acceptable foods, it can be quite a learning experience.

There are gluten-free and sugar-free cake and bread mixes available on store shelves now, along with sugar-free frostings. Just keep in mind these still have fats, carbohydrates, and calories that can pack on the weight if not consumed in moderation. There are alternatives to chocolate for cooking, and other choices to look at as well. If it is recommended by your physician to eliminate all meat except fish and some sea foods from your diet, you would need to look at other protein sources such as mushrooms, eggs, yogurt, beans, legumes, etc., especially if you do not care for fish or seafood. Shrimp cooked in a wok with vegetables and rice or pasta makes an excellent meal. This can also be a wonderful meal with no shrimp, but use a stir fry sauce for season-ing, or whatever your favorite seasoning may be such as lemon and garlic, chili flavored sauce, or your favorite spice. The choices are only limited by your imagination. The vegetables can be anything you are allowed in your diet such as fresh spinach, tomatoes, onion, garlic, broccoli, brussel sprouts, cauliflower, green beans, squash, okra, radishes, and the list goes on. Fresh or frozen is best for lower sodium, but canned vegetables can be purchased now with low sodium content. And there again, dur-ing gardening season, your local farmers market is a good source of fresh produce usually at great prices.

For low kidney function diets see the list of low po-tassium and low phosphate foods, toward the back of this book, to help make better food choices.

My husband Jim, will teasingly make comments about food commercials on television, but he does not cheat on his diet restrictions because he wants to achieve and maintain improvement in his kidney function to continue his efforts toward his goal of never having to go on kidney dialysis. Between the trip to Thailand for stem cell treatments, and the changes in diet recommended by the Thai physicians, Jim's kidney function has improved from 16 to 22%.

It takes establishing your mindset toward your goal to remember that food is a necessity for life, and can be made very tasteful with little effort. One of the big hurdles is to stop focusing on the foods you are not to have, and start imagining all the possibilities to spice up the foods you can have.

There are some significant "do not eat or drink foods and liquids" such as dairy and most dairy products, chocolate, nuts, corn, carrots, brown rice, sticky rice, avocado, apricots, etc. There will be a list in the back of the book.

As stated before, there are people who are not, or do not have to be so strict with their diet, and they get improvement in kidney function while others continue to decline.

CHAPTER 10

꙳꙳꙳

CHANGING; NOT ENOUGH TO NOW EMPOWERED

As Jim and I continue this journey for his health so he can maintain a better quality of life, I continue to teach Jim about his disease processes, exercise, nutrition, medications, resources for researching new information, and questions to ask his healthcare providers.

In previous chapters, we discussed not enough of many things. In today's world, we have the power of the Internet, access to healthcare providers, and many public libraries for information gathering, to include providing for the learning needs of the hearing and vision impaired.

What we haven't achieved in many areas is providing

the needed information to those with poor reading skills (a form of information that can be referred back to, not just verbalizing the information), and overcoming the old notion that "we can't question a doctor".

Everyone needs to feel empowered enough to ask their doctor questions, and to not feel they will be ridiculed if they asked for whatever they need to enhance their learning such as a DVD or CD instead of written materials. The information packet, given to renal patients is usually too much, and too overpowering for information retention. Not to mention, there are usually other important priorities or worries in a person's life, on any given day.

On the journey to empowering yourself with more confidence, through the process of gaining knowledge, it is important to remain respectful of your healthcare providers. It is better not to bounce from one physician to another simply because you don't agree with him/her. You can ask questions, state your disagreement, ask if there is an alternative treatment or medication, and be able to tell your doctor what your healthcare goals are. If you're being treated by a team of healthcare providers such as your primary care physician, nephrologist, cardiologist, etc., always provide an updated medication and treatment list to each one as you have an appointment. If we want to hold our healthcare providers responsible for their role in treating us, we must hold ourselves responsible for our role in being part of the healthcare team. Being empowered and becoming a member of the team responsible for your health is an essential component to the outcome of your overall well-being.

I encourage you to actively participate in the decision-making processes regarding treatment choices and options for your healthcare. Many of you feel your doctor is so busy and does not have time to listen to your questions or concerns. I recommend you write your questions and/or concerns on paper and hand it to your physician when he or she enters the treatment room (if in his office setting), or when you see the doctor at the dialysis clinic during his regular visit with you since this is when the doctor assesses your care, treatment plan, labs, and orders.

Doctors are human, so don't be afraid to voice your questions and/or concerns and be honest about any symptoms you may be experiencing, especially if you are on dialysis because the dialysate solution may need to be adjusted, which requires an order from your doctor.

Ask your doctor if there are any dietary changes you need to make based on your lab results, or if he/she is going to change any medication orders. All symptoms should be reported to your doctor and dialysis team (if this applies). Report symptoms such as swelling, shortness of breath, increased weakness, pain, cramping, episodes of chest pain, emergency room visits or hospitalizations and reasons, nausea or vomiting, changes in bowel or bladder habits, fever, etc. Also report to your doctor any injuries, changes in caregiver support systems at home, medication changes made by other doctors, (it is best to bring the medicine bottle with you so it can be reviewed by your dialysis team), and any new diagnosis you may have.

Medicare and many health insurance companies are now promoting free annual wellness visits to your physician. Medicare has a toll free number 1-800-MED-ICAR for information, Oklahoma Medicaid information can be reached by dialing 2-1-1, and you can check with your private insurance company for their toll free number for information, and many of them have a toll free nurse line available 24 hours per day 7 days per week.

For most vulnerable citizens, we healthcare professionals must advocate for them, provide them or their families/caregivers with the knowledge and resources to contact so they have access to entities that can meet their healthcare needs.

Many people are fearful and questioning of the Health Care Reform Act, or Obama care, as it is being referred to. It is a dance, not so graceful right now, between our government, that is supposed to be for the people, and we citizens. Empowering ourselves with knowledge is going to be the key to positive healthcare outcomes.

CHAPTER 11

❧

EMPOWERED TO MAKE YOU THE PRIORITY

Jim's physicians did not threaten to discontinue Jim as a patient when we discussed treatment options and expressed thoughts of pursuing stem cell treatments outside the United States. You know you have aligned with the right health care team when all concerns about your health and treatment options can be discussed openly and honestly without negative repercussions.

Of course, we can't ask a health care provider to discuss options that are not legal. However, there are herbal, natural, and alternative therapeutic treatment modalities, not approved by the FDA, and not utilized by the mainstream medical professionals.

Acupuncture, pressure neutralization therapy, reflexology, massage therapy, herbology, and naturopathy are all treatment modalities growing in popularity, and some of these are even being covered by more forward thinking health insurance companies that are focusing on prevention and wellness versus always treating symptoms of injuries or disease processes without ever returning a person to a state of well-being.

In my opinion, these are things that have resulted in many Americans living on disability rather than achieving a state of wellness that would have allowed them to return to work.

Being empowered to make YOU the priority means deciding what treatment options are out there, and which ones will work best for you. These are the areas where health care reform may not be beneficial, as health insurance companies are not always on board for alternative treatment options. This amazes me as many cancer treatment centers and addiction rehab centers now use acupuncture as part of the overall treatment processes toward healing/curing a person, but we go to an acupuncturist for pain management or other health concerns and it is cash or credit card for payment. We can receive massage therapy in a chiropractor's office and some insurance companies will cover part of the cost as an overall part of the treatment. Don't get me wrong, these are wonderful things happening, we just need more of it to truly allow people options.

CHAPTER 12

꒰ᔶ꒱

THE GIFT OF BETTER HEALTH
OUR JOURNEY TO THAILAND

Jim was diagnosed with Stage IV Chronic Kidney Disease on October 18, 2010. Although he has Type II insulin-dependent diabetes mellitus, Jim has always been healthy, and just did not go to the doctor unless he had to. He worked hard and felt good. It was time for my annual trek to the doctor for my checkup, and I encouraged Jim to allow me to make him an appointment for an annual checkup. I explained to Jim that as a diabetic, he should have a minimum of an annual checkup with his physician. During his checkup, the physician told Jim he had not been seen in a long while and no labs had been done in a long time either. We were both shocked when his physician called and told Jim his kidney function was at 23%, his creatinine and BUN were high, and he needed to see a nephrologist as soon as possible. I had Jim give his doctor the name of a well-known nephrologist in Tahlequah, Oklahoma. The referral was made, and we saw a partner of the nephrologist we had requested as the one the referral was sent to was out of town. Jim agreed to see the other nephrologist, and she right away wanted to do a CAT scan with contrast to Jim's kidneys to make a differential diagnosis of the cause of the kidney disease. She told us this would more than likely put Jim into complete renal failure and dialysis would have to be started. We told her we would have to think about that. She set up the appointment for the scan, and two days prior to the test, I called and cancelled the test, with Jim's agreement. We saw the partner nephrologist one more time, and informed her we cancelled the CT scan. I asked her if she would consider an ultrasound of the kidneys. She agreed and it was done. We notified the office we wanted to see the nephrologist we originally requested. That appointment was set up by the receptionist, and Jim has had all his appointments with him since that time.

I was already researching renal/diabetic diets and had made changes to our way of eating. During this time, I had contacted Julia, a dietitian I had worked with for several years. We made an appointment and consulted with her over a four-month time frame. She was a wonderful resource and guide. The nephrologist did not agree with the supplements the dietician had Jim taking and requested Jim stop them.

During our first visit with the requested nephrologist of our choice, he reviewed the ultrasound results with us, and there was a small mass on Jim's right kidney. We opted to leave it alone and have a new ultrasound in October to see if the mass had enlarged at all. During this visit, we were given a large manila envelope and told, "There is some good information and recipes in there, and it would be better if you didn't have dairy products." The nephrologist determined Jim's kidney disease was more caused by blood pressure in the low end of the high range undetected for long time, rather than his diabetes. Oh, and the first set of complete labs ordered by the nephrologist cost us $1200. The nephrologist requested that no medicine be taken by Jim without his approval as he would know if his kidneys could handle it. We agreed to this. Jim told his nephrologist that his goal was to do whatever was necessary to not start kidney dialysis.

Jim has a basic set of labs drawn every month that

includes a renal panel, CBC, and UA so we can monitor his status and know how to adjust our diet as needed. We continue to do this and the lab results show us if we are eating foods higher in phosphates, potassium, etc. One problem with the renal diet is the difficulty in eating enough iron rich foods. Last year when Jim's red blood cell count, white blood cell count, and hematocrit started dropping, then his total iron binding capacity dropped, I started researching again. The nephrologist likes to have IV iron infusions as needed, and Jim did not want this if it could be avoided. I know that regular iron tablets do not work for renal patients, so I found "food source liquid iron" supplement. This is very absorbable and does not cause gastric distress of any kind in most people. Jim started on that last fall, and continues to take 10 ML every morning. It works for him, as his labs are staying within normal ranges.

As we journeyed through all this, Jim's kidney function continued to decline. During all our research, we would run across all the wonderful treatments being performed overseas. We read about stem cells, kidney transplants, islet cell transplants, and other treatment modalities. During this time, our friend ask about stem cell treatments for his 10-year-old grandson with a diagnosis of Common Variable Immune Deficiency. I researched this and emailed him information of who, where, how, etc. on treatments being done overseas, which he shared with his daughter and son-in-law. I would tell/read to Jim about what I found, and would then read to him about what is being done with kidney disease also. In December, 2012, I asked Jim if I could send a query to the doctors in Thailand. I chose to send this to www.thaimedicalvacation.com as they work with multiple physician groups, and assist with all travel plans, hotel arrangements, and transport to and from treatments, etc. After we heard back, Jim's kidney function was at 18%, then in February and March 2013 he was at 16%. It seemed that no matter what we did, the GFR would not come up. And believe me, we were sticking to a strict diet. At that point, I told Jim if we were going to try other options, we needed to do so prior to dialysis, which is usually started when the kidney function is at 15% or less. Jim had his left wrist Cimino fistula placed in June, 2011 in case of a crisis or emergency need for dialysis since the risk of death goes up 40% if they have to use a central line for access to administer dialysis.

After our appointment with Jim's nephrologist on March 15, 2013, Jim made the decision that we could actively pursue going to Thailand. We had spoken with the nephrologist during Jim's appointment about stem cell treatments for Jim, and he was all for it, and stated that Thailand had the most sophisticated program and success. He told us he could not take an official stance on this as it is not done here in the U.S. as a routine form of FDA approved treatment. The stem cell treatments in the U.S. are being done in clinical trials, radiation is used to wipe out your immune system, and if you survive the first year, you should make it.

We contacted www.thaimedicalvacation.com, and confirmed our desire for Jim to have treatments. They sent us a treatment plan for Jim after their physicians reviewed his medical records that we scanned and emailed to them. The Thai New Year holiday was to occur during the time we were to be in Thailand, so their hotel arrangements for us changed three times. I called my oldest son, Scottlee, as I knew he had been to Bangkok several times in his travels. He called that night and made us reservations at the Marriott Langsuan in Bangkok, Thailand. Of course, we had to come up with the money for all this to the tune of $30,000 which would include Jim's medical treatments, our travel there and back, hotel, and food. My friend Helen put it all into perspective. She said, if you needed a new vehicle, you would not think twice about signing a $30,000 note. And, she was right! We refinanced our home, got a great fixed interest rate, and in four days prior to closing, the bank called and stated they wanted the siding redone and completely finished by Monday, April 1 before closing papers were signed. That was Easter weekend. To get this done, our friends pitched in, and it was done! Of course, by this time, Jim's endurance had become very low because of the low kidney function. He was usually able to work about three hours per day before he was exhausted.

We flew out on April 5, 2013, to Dallas, San Francisco, then to Hong Kong and finally on to Bangkok. I had arranged for us an escort through all the airports due to security checks, customs, etc. as we only had two hours on the ground between every flight. That can get a little harried. And of course, Jim's endurance at that point was not good.

We were in Bangkok for 22 days. Jim received three stem cell treatments, three kidney fresh cell injections, six acupuncture treatments, and three peptide injections. He received a total of 10 million stem cells overall. They changed our diet even more by instructing Jim not to eat any meat except fish and some seafood, cook all vegetables, no sticky rice, no brown rice, no white breads, no corn or carrots, no coconut milk, and no dairy except for yogurt, if desired. Jim was to have only one cup of coffee a day, and then water or green tea. Jim drinks rice milk, as he says it tastes more like "real" milk than any of them. I reviewed all the complete protein plant foods, and most of them Jim is not allowed to eat such as beans, legumes, etc.

We returned home on April 30, 2013 and had Jim's labs drawn on May 1st for his appointment with the nephrologist on May 3rd. His kidney function was up to 18%. Jim's lab results on June 6th showed 22% kidney function. The physicians in Thailand attribute both the stem cell treatments, and the diet changes to the success. They expect improvement for a total of six months.

God opened all these doors, and had it all fall in place. And we are believing that Jim will be able to maintain his goal of no dialysis.

CHAPTER 13

❦

FOLLOW-UP
ONE YEAR AFTER STEM CELL TREATMENT

Jim's kidney function improved from 16% to 22% within one month of receiving stem cell treatments and acupuncture in Thailand, in April, 2013. His GFR continues to fluctuate between 19 and 22% on the monthly lab results. One of the most challenging aspects of our diet is to keep Jim's iron levels within normal limits. It is difficult to eat enough iron rich foods that are allowed on a renal diet. We eat a great deal of fresh spinach in everything. I have started taking a daily dose of food source liquid iron, and Jim takes this twice a day now.

Jim is now on four different blood pressure medications

to control his blood pressure in a range below 140/80. The important thing is to control the blood pressure, and it is a bit of an oxymoron. The kidney disease causes the blood pressure to go up, and an elevated blood pressure, left untreated, can cause continued deterioration of the kidney function.

During this past year, I have been reading Dr. Mark Stengler's e-news letters and printed health newsletters. I shared with Jim the information about new studies and research, etc. we called and arranged a telephone consult with Dr. Stengler on February 14, 2014. We were asked to email a health history, lab results, medication list, names of Jim's primary care and specialty physicians, and any other pertinent information regarding Jim's health for Dr. Stengler to review prior to the consult. Dr. Stengler is an NM.D. and naturopathist with a large clinic in Encinita, California. He recommended Renadyl, Glutithione, Fish Oil Plus, and Nattokinase for Jim. The surprise for us was the Renadyl. Dr. Stengler informed us the Renadyl had to be ordered from www.renadyl.com, and this product was specifically developed for Stage III and Stage IV chronic kidney disease patients. It is a probiotic that is coated to withstand stomach acid so the active ingredients (probiotic strains) are not released until they reach the intestines. There are several probiotic brands that do this, but Renadyl specifically targets the nitrogenous toxins that normally get absorbed into the bloodstream to be taken to the liver and kidneys for filtering. The Renadyl neutralizes and attaches to the toxins while they are there in the intestine, and these are eliminated through the bowel, thus taking a great deal of work off the kidneys.

Jim recently told his family and friends that he feels better than he has since Christmas of 2013. Jim said he felt good at that time, but he could tell the toxins in his system were starting to affect his energy and endurance again. Jim has been on the new natural/herbal medicines, that Dr. Stengler ordered, for two weeks, and he can already tell the difference.

We continue to adhere to a strict diabetic, no added salt, renal diet with no meats except fish and some seafood. Jim maintains a healthy weight that flucuates between 174 and 177 pounds with his height at 5 feet 9 inches. We have successfully stayed the course for 3 1/2 years, and Jim's goal continues to be "no dialysis".

ALTERNATIVE SUBSTITUTIONS WHEN COOKING

USE	INSTEAD OF
1 1/2 cups ground rolled oats	1 cup sifted wheat flour
3/4 cup coarse cornmeal	1 cup sifted wheat flour
1/2 tablespoon cornstarch	1 tablespoon flour
Rice or almond milk	Dairy milk
1 Tbspn vinegar in 1 cup rice or almond milk	1 cup buttermilk or sour cream
1 1/8 cup butter or margarine	1 cup vegetable shortening
Carob powder	Cocoa powder or chocolate
3 Tbspn carob powder + 1 Tbspn butter	1 ounce chocolate
1 cup Sugarfree honey or sugar-free syrup	1 cup sugar
1 cup Splenda	1 cup sugar
1 cup sugar free honey	1 cup light Karo or corn syrup
2 Tbspn peanut butter extract flavoring	1/4 cup peanut butter
1/2 cup no sugar added applesauce	1/2 cup butter
Rice or gluten-free pasta	Regular pasta
Almond or rice flour	White or wheat flour

POTASSIUM RESTRICTED DIET GUIDELINES

POTASSIUM RICH FOODS TO AVOID

Chocolate, molasses, nuts, salt substitutes, apricots, avocado, cantaloupe, honeydew melon, nectarines, plantain, tangelos, artichokes, butter beans, yams, dried peas, beans, lentils, baked potatoes, commercial fries and chips, sweet potatoes, Swiss chard, tomato paste/puree, winter squash

POTASSIUM RICH FOODS TO LIMIT ONE SERVING PER DAY

FRUITS

1/2 medium banana
3/4 cup BlackBerries
1 cup boysenberries
12 cherries
1 medium pear
2 medium plums
1 cup prune juice
1/2 grapefruit
1 medium kiwi fruit
1 cup mulberries

3/4 cup mandarin oranges
1/2 cup orange juice
1 medium orange
1 medium peach
2 figs
3 prunes
2 tablespoon raisins
1 cup Raspberries
1 1/4 cups strawberries
1 1/4 cup watermelon

POTASSIUM RICH FOODS TO LIMIT

VEGETABLES

ONE SERVING EQUALS 1/2 CUP PER DAY

Asparagus	beets	brussels sprouts
collard greens	corn	cow peas
dandelion greens	kale	mushrooms
mixed vegetables	parsnips	pumpkin
potato leached	spinach	turnips
tomato juice	canned tomatoes	zucchini

*All potatoes should be leached before they are cooked. Peel the potatoes and cut into small pieces. Cover completely with water, and soak in the refrigerator for at least four hours. Drain well and cook in fresh water. Leaching potatoes will remove much of the potassium.

Limit dairy to 1/2 cup per day if you continue to use

PREFERABLE FOODS TO CONSUME

Rice or almond milk   nondairy creamer

cream cheese or   sherbet or frozen fruit pops
cottage cheese

broth or water based soups

refined grains such as white bread, crackers, cereals, rice and pasta

refined white dinner rolls, bagels, English muffins, or croissants

green peas/canned or   green beans or wax beans
frozen

leached potatoes	rutabaga	winter squash
cabbage	beets	carrots
celery	cucumbers	eggplant
lettuce	peppers	onions
tomatoes	summer squash	
Beef	pork	lamb

poultry and fish

EXCEPT no organ meats, walleye, Pollack, or sardine fish

USE: butter, margarine, mayonnaise, salad dressings, shortenings, vegetable oils

INSTEAD OF: Cream including fat free, half-and-half, sesame butter, or sour cream

PREFERABLE FOOD CHOICES

LOW SODIUM, DIABETIC, RENAL DIET
(low potassium, phosphorus, Limited protein)

SPICES

Greek seasoning no salt added	black pepper	garlic powder
lemon pepper	turmeric	cinnamon

MEAT

Farm raised cat Fish	shrimp	crabmeat
veggie meats (soy free whenever possible)		

VEGETABLES

Green beans	broccoli	cauliflower
bell peppers	onions	tomatoes
yellow squash	zucchini	okra
fresh spinach	romaine lettuce	celery

FRUITS

Apples	pineapple	strawberries
blueberries	watermelon	

OTHER

Rice or almond milk
oatmeal
white rice / no sticky rice
mustard
butter or margarine
safflower, sunflower, or olive oil
eggs
pasta, gluten-free preferable

RECIPES

ANGEL HAIR PASTA WITH SHRIMP AND CRABMEAT

APPLE CRISP

BACON and SAUSAGE LINGUINE

BACON—SPINACH QUICHE

BROCCOLI and RICE CASSEROLE

CHEESE FREE BREAKFAST PIZZA

HOMEMADE SLAW

LOW CARB BREAD

NO BAKE COOKIES

OVEN FRIED FISH NUGGETS

SQUASH FRITTERS

TASTY GREEN BEANS

ZUCCHINI BREAD

ANGEL HAIR PASTA WITH SHRIMP AND CRAB MEAT

2 tablespoons olive oil
1 cup small cooked frozen
  shrimp
1/2 cup flaky imitation
  crab meat
1/2 cup chopped broccoli
1/2 cup chopped
  cauliflower

1/2 cup chopped red bell
  pepper
1 teaspoon garlic powder
1 teaspoon basil
1 teaspoon chives
1/4 cup finely grated
  veggie cheese
12 ounces angel hair pasta
  gluten free

Place 1 tablespoon oil in large skillet. Add shrimp and crab meat and cook over medium heat until heated through. Remove from skillet. Cook pasta in large pan of boiling water with 1 tablespoon oil added to prevent boiling over. Rinse pasta in colander under hot water after cooked. In large skillet add 1 tablespoon oil, all vegetables, and all seasonings. Cook about 6 to 8 minutes. Add shrimp and crab meat. Place cooked, rinsed pasta in large bowl, add shrimp mixture, cover with grated cheese.

APPLE CRISP

---

5 cups sliced, peeled   3/4 cup oats
  apples   1 teaspoon cinnamon
1 cup Splenda brown sugar 1/2 cup butter
3/4 cup flour

NOTE: for gluten-free use rice, almond, or oat flour.

Combine brown sugar, flour, oats, cinnamon, and melted butter. Place apples in rectangle baking dish. Pat combine ingredients over top of apples. Bake at 425° for 45 minutes.

BACON AND SAUSAGE LINGUINE

16 ounces linguine pasta (regular or gluten-free)

12 ounces veggie sausage

4 slices veggie bacon

1 1/4 cups water

1/2 cup finely chopped red bell pepper

2 tablespoons pure lemon juice

1/2 cup diced tomatoes

1/2 teaspoon Greek seasoning (sodium free)

1/4 teaspoon garlic powder

1/4 teaspoon black pepper

Cook linguine pasta in large pot of boiling water with 1 tablespoon olive oil in the water. In a large skillet cook the bacon, then the sausage. Cut/crumble the bacon and sausage into small bits. Cook the bacon, sausage, water, and seasonings in the large skillet until liquid is reduced by half. Stir in lemon juice, red pepper, and tomatoes. Pour the sauce over linguine pasta to serve.

BACON–SPINACH QUICHE

One pie crust
8 slices cooked, crumbled
  veggie bacon
1 small chopped onion
1 cup fresh spinach
4 eggs
2 teaspoons olive oil

2 cups half-and-half or
  nondairy cream
1/4 teaspoon sea salt
1/4 teaspoon pepper
1/4 teaspoon Greek
  seasoning
1 cup shredded veggie
  cheese

Preheat oven to 425°. Place uncooked pie dough in deep pie plate, cover with aluminum foil and bake 10 minutes, remove foil and bake three more minutes. Reduce oven temperature to 325°. Cook bacon, crumble. Cook onion and spinach in 2 teaspoons olive oil. Mix in Greek seasoning, sea salt, and pepper. In large bowl, beat eggs with fork and then beat in cream. Sprinkle bacon, onion and spinach mixture, and cheese in the pie crust. Gently pour egg mixture over this. Bake 45 to 50 minutes or until knife inserted in center comes out clean. Let stand 10 minutes before serving.

BROCCOLI AND RICE CASSEROLE

One small diced onion
1/4 cup melted butter
2 cups quick cooking rice
2 cups water
one can cream of
  mushroom soup
1/2 teaspoon sea salt

1 cup shredded veggie
  cheese
2 – 10 ounce bags frozen
  broccoli
cornflake crumbs browned
  in butter

Combine all ingredients except cornflake crumbs. Cook in crockpot, covered, on low heat 7 to 10 hours. Just before serving, sprinkle cornflake crumbs over top.

CHEESE FREE BREAKFAST PIZZA

Chopped, diced vegetables of choice such as onion, mushrooms, garlic, black olives, tomatoes, etc.
Cooked and crumbled veggie bacon

Cooked and chopped veggie sausage
8 eggs
Greek seasoning sodium free
garlic powder
black pepper

MORNAY SAUCE

Melt 2 tablespoons butter in saucepan. Whisk in 2 tablespoons all-purpose flour until smooth. Cook for two minutes whisking continuously. Gradually whisk in 1 cup half-and-half or Nondairy cream substitute. Continue whisking 3 to 5 minutes or until thickened. Remove from heat and whisk in Greek seasoning, sea salt, and pepper.

Spread Mornay sauce over pizza shaped dough of choice, may use gluten-free, sprinkle vegetables over this, crack open and place eggs for eight pieces of pizza. Bake at 425° 20 to 25 minutes.

HOME MADE SLAW

3/4 cup Crisco

1 cup apple cider

2 tablespoon Splenda
sugar

Combine these ingredients and bring to boil.

POUR OVER

one head shredded
   cabbage

3/4 cup Splenda sugar

one large diced onion

1 tablespoon celery seed

one diced green pepper,
   optional

dash of sea salt

Mix well. Refrigerate overnight before serving.

LOW CARB BREAD

1/2 cup rice or whey
  protein powder
2 teaspoons baking
  powder

1/4 cup almond butter
1/4 cup sugar free honey
4 eggs

Mix dry ingredients. In a separate bowl beat butter until creamy. Add honey and beat about one minute. Add one egg at a time; beat after each egg added. Then add dry ingredients. Bake at 300° for 40 minutes.

*If you use vanilla flavored protein powder –it makes a great low-carb cake.

NO BAKE COOKIES

3 cups Splenda sugar
1/2 cup butter or
  margarine
4 tablespoons carob
  powder
1/2 cup rice or almond
  milk

6 cups quick cooking
  oatmeal
2 teaspoons vanilla
1 tablespoon peanut butter
  flavored extract optional

Combine butter, milk, sugar, and carob powder in large pan over high heat. When mixture reaches full boil, continue cooking at full boil for five minutes, stirring constantly. Remove from burner, add vanilla, peanut butter flavor extract, and oatmeal. Mix well. Drop by teaspoonful onto wax paper, and allow cookies to set up. When cookies are completely cool, place in baking dish with wax paper between layers and refrigerate. Makes three dozen cookies.

OVEN FRIED FISH NUGGETS

1/3 cup rice crumbs
1/3 cup crushed rice chex
1/2 teaspoon sea salt
1/4 teaspoon pepper
3 tablespoons finely grated
  veggie cheese

1 1/2 pounds catfish fillets
  cut into 1 inch cubes
butter flavored cooking
  spray

In a shallow dish combine the rice crumbs, rice chex, grated cheese, salt, and pepper. Spray fish with butter flavored cooking spray and roll in crumb mixture. Place on baking sheet coated with cooking spray. Bake at 375° for 15 to 20 minutes.

SQUASH FRITTERS

1 cup grated yellow squash
1 egg beaten
1 teaspoon Splenda
3 tablespoons flour

1 teaspoon melted butter, oil
2 tablespoons finely chopped onion
black pepper to taste

Mix all ingredients together in bowl. Spoon into large skillet (heated) with small amount of oil. Pat down to form patties, and fry until browned on both sides.

TASTY GREEN BEANS

1 pound fresh or frozen
   green beans
2 teaspoons butter
3 large finely chopped
   green onions
1/2 teaspoon Splenda

1/2 teaspoon Greek
   seasoning, sodium free
1/4 teaspoon black pepper
1/4 teaspoon garlic powder
2 tablespoons grated fresh
   lemon
1/4 teaspoon basil

Bring 1/2 inch water to boil in 10 inch covered skillet. Add green beans; cover; cook over medium to low heat about eight minutes. Drain in colander. Heat butter in skillet over medium heat. Add green onions and Splenda; cook about two minutes. Add Greek seasoning, black pepper, garlic powder, basil, and grated lemon. Stir in green beans. Cook about two minutes or until heated through.

ZUCCHINI BREAD

3 eggs beaten
1 cup cooking oil
2 cup Splenda
1 teaspoon baking soda
3 cups Zucchini peeled
and shredded
2 teaspoons vanilla
1/4 teaspoon baking
powder

1 teaspoon sea salt
3 teaspoons cinnamon
1/2 cup walnuts optional
3 cups flour, rice or
almond flour for
gluten-free
*may change cooking oil
to 1 cup unsweetened
applesauce

Combine oil or applesauce, Splenda, and zucchini. Add to well beaten eggs and mix well. Add vanilla. Sift dry ingredients together. Add dry, sifted ingredients to zucchini mixture. Bake at 325° for one hour in loaf pans.

RESOURCES

Hogan, R. D., Joan Brookhyser; The Vegetarian Diet For Kidney Disease, 2010, Basic Health Publications, Inc.

Journal of the American Society of Nephrology 08 – 01 – 2012. Volume 23 no. 8, 1291 – 1298. Reimbursement of Dialysis: A Comparison of Seven Countries. Raymond van holder, Andrew Davenport, Thierry Hannedouche, Jersen Kooman, Andreas Kribben, Norbert Lamiere, Gerhard Lonnemann, Peter Magner, David , Mendelssohn, Subodh J. Sogg, Rachel N. Shaffer, Sharon M. Moe, Wim Van Biesen, Frank van der Sande, Rajnish Mehrotra, and on be-half of the Dialysis Advisory Group of the American Society of Nephrology.

Kallenbach, Judith Z.; Review of Hemodialysis for Nurses and Dialysis Personnel. Eighth Edition 2012, Elseviar, Inc. Mosby,Inc.

Kee, Joyce LeFever; Prentice-Hall Handbook of Laboratory and Diagnostic Test with Nursing

Implications; Sixth Edition, 2009, Pearson Prentice Hall.

Kolbe, RD, CSR, LD, Nina. Kidney Health Gourmet Cookbook. Third Edition, September 6, 2013.

Lippincott Manual of Nursing Practice, Third Edition, JB Lippincott Company, Philadelphia, Pennsylvania, 1982.

Nettina, Sandra M., Lippincott Manual of Nursing Practice 10th edition, Lippincott Williams and Wilkins, June, 2013.

Philip, Richard B., Herbal—Drug Interactions and Adverse Effects: An Evidenced-Based Quick Reference Guide, McGraw-Hill, 2004.

Sriwatanakul, M.D., PhD, Kampon, Phoenix Rejuvenation Center, Bangkok, Thailand.

Stengler, NMD, Mark , Stengler Center for Integrative Medicine. Encinita, California.

Stengler NMD, Mark. Natural Healing Library, 2013, New Market Health Publishing, LLC.

The National Kidney Foundation, Inc. 30 E. 33rd St., New York, NY 10016. 800 – 622 – 9010. kidney.org

Touchette, PhD, Nancy; American Diabetes Association Complete Guide to Diabetes; 4th Edition, 2005.

White, Linda B., The Herbal Drug Store, Rodale Press, August 1, 2000.

Special thanks and gratitude to our four wonderful children, Josh, Scottlee, Melissa, and Tony, family, and many friends. A very special praise goes to our friends, Brenda Nixon, R.N. for her proofreading and editing talents, and to Helen Alewine, R.N. for her continued, endearing, positive support. To Jim's physicians, and all the professional persons we have encountered along the way. Our journey and this book would not have been possible without all of you.